Sex: The 15 Best Sex Tips and Tricks That Will Greatly Impress Your Partner and Enhance Your Sex Life Forever

# Table of Contents

# Intro

Congratulations on your desire to impress your partner and enhance your sex life!

There are few topics as taboo to discuss as sex. In fact, it is so taboo, that it isn't even listed when people talk about what topics should never be discussed in public (that's left to religion and politics). Our conservative society discourages honest and frank conversations about sex. Instead, individuals are left to watch pornographic movies and are lead to believe THAT is how everyone is doing it. Alternatively, they try to stick to being good little boys and girls and stay focused on just having basic sex that inevitably leaves both partners unfulfilled and unsatisfied. Following that plan, though, individuals often go without knowing what it is that their partners want and/or need when it comes to sex. One of the number one reasons couples stop having regular sex is because the passion dies and it become boring and monotonous. It's a chore instead of a pleasure.

What if there was another way? What if it were possible to bring sex out of the closet and really appreciate it for the many benefits, both for mental and physical health, that great sex can provide? What if you could learn the tips and tricks that would impress your partner and revive the passion and excitement you once had? Individuals could then strive to improve their experiences and creating a scenario that would enhance their sex lives for the rest of their lives.

In this book, you will first learn some of the basic tips and tricks to impress your partner and improve your sexual experience. This foundation is critical to getting all the rest just right. It is the little things that tend to be most impressive because it shows that you care enough to pay attention to every detail.

In the second part of this guide, you will learn some tips and tricks that you can explore with your partner to enhance your sex life and add some new passion and excitement. Be open to exploring the different tips even if it is just about starting a conversation. You never know where it might lead.

There are no limits on what you might discover about yourself and your partner when you aim to impress. Have fun with it and see where it takes you!

# Part 1
# The Basics

# Confidence Is The Key

Sex is about more than just how you look. Confidence is the number one thing you can do to impress your partner and improve your sex life. Most individuals experience moments when they aren't feeling as confident as they'd like to. For some, this is more than a fleeting moment. It is closer to a constant state of mind. However, having confidence in your body and sexuality is a huge turn on for both men and women and makes the sexual experience that much more exciting.

We will never be as pretty, skinny, strong, young, voluptuous, hung or handsome as the next guy or gal. Having confidence isn't about how you look. It's about how you choose to feel.

Fortunately, it is possible to improve your confidence in the bedroom by becoming more comfortable with your sexual side. When you know you are good at doing something, you have more confidence in yourself.

Here are a few tips on how to improve your own confidence in the bedroom:

## Explore Your Own Body

Whether you are male or female, the more you know about your body, the better you will feel and the more confidence you will have. Learn what you like and don't like before sharing that with your partner. What areas do you like touched and which ones are off limits because they just don't feel good? Be sure to be adventurous with your exploration and don't be afraid to touch places you've only ever touched with a wash cloth.

## Explore What Others Are Doing

The more you know about sex, the more confident you feel. Reading this book is a great start, but don't stop here. Don't be afraid to watch some porn, read sex magazines and erotic fiction or to check out some group discussions around sex. While not everyone is going to do things the way they do in the movies, it can give you some knowledge and new ideas to explore.

Society often discourages positive feelings around sex and most families don't discuss it at all. Fortunately, you can decide to get more information on your own and learn what you've been missing.

## Take Steps to Look Better

Do some push ups to pump yourself up. Put on some sexy lingerie. Dim the lights (but don't go totally dark). These are just a few of the things you can do to feel better about the way you look.

Just remember, it's not about how you look but about how you feel. If you feel good, your partner will notice and it will be a big turn on!

# Personal Grooming Matters

It seems like it would be obvious to take care of personal grooming before jumping into bed with your partner but this is one of those areas where we often get comfortable or even just lazy in long term relationships. If you are well groomed, you will be much more appealing in the bedroom! But what does well groomed mean?

Different people have different opinions of what is well groomed. However, there are certain standards that everyone agrees upon.

- Showered and clean - If you've just come from the gym or working in the yard, it isn't likely to entice anyone to jump into the sack with you. Be sure to wash all your parts, especially if you want them to be explored later! Sure, sweaty sex can be fun on occasion but not as a routine.

- Shaving - Knowing what your partner likes helps you to know just how much shaving you need to do. Some women hate facial hair and tend to get "burned" if there is any stubble when their man goes down on them to take care of business. On the other hand, some men like a bit of a landing strip and think it's very sexy. Be sure to honor your partner's desires in this area if you want to really impress.

- Hands and feet - Don't make the mistake of having your partner be cut by a sharp finger nail or find a foot full of nasty calluses. Be sure to have clean, trimmed nails and feet that are soft and callous free for maximum exploration.

- Cleaning "down there" - Whether you are male or female, it needs to be said that some care should be taken to make sure your genital area (front and back) are clean and ready to receive.

- Go easy on scents - Some scents can be overpowering and a turn off. Others can leave a residue that can be a turn off if one is kissing or licking certain body parts. Stick to a light scent sprayed on the hair for best results.

- Brush your teeth - There's nothing worse than kissing someone with bad breath. And, while you are at it, make sure to brush your tongue as a lot of the odor resides on the buildup found on the tongue.

- Lotion up - No, that's not lube up, that comes later. Both men and women like soft skin. Make sure yours isn't dry and scaly but using some lotion before you get to business.

You don't have to spend hours grooming every time you plan to have sex with your partner, however, if you want to make it a special occasion, take the extra time.

# Foreplay All Day

If you want to go above and beyond impressing your partner in the bedroom, then begin foreplay as soon as you wake up in the morning! No, that doesn't mean you should start sex first thing in the morning (although that's not always a bad thing). Foreplay is about more than what you do just before engaging in sex. The brain is the largest sex organ in the human body. This means that sex is about more than just the visual and kinesthetic aspects we all know and love. Site and touch play only a small part in the overall experience of having a great sex life.

Think about what it was like when you were dating. You often sent notes via text or email all day long telling your partner how special they are to you. You may have dropped little hints about how much you find them attractive or how excited you get just thinking of them. These acts often get forgotten as couples get busy with their everyday lives and fall into a pattern of comfort with one another. However, to really spice things up and have a great sex life well into your old age, think foreplay all day.

What, then, are some things you can do to focus on foreplay throughout the day?

- Sharing a passionate kiss before you each rush off to your busy days at work.
- Going out of the way to make sure your partner feels good about him/herself.
- Doing things that will take some of the pressure and stress off your partner whether that's running an extra errand on your way home from work or taking out the trash.
- Being interested in (but not jealous of) what your partner is doing when you aren't around.
- Remembering to check your baggage at the door. Sometimes partners will come home with so much stress from work that their significant other will assume that tonight isn't a good night and skip the obvious ques. The more you are able to leave your work stress at work, the better the foreplay will be.
- Foreplay all day touch shouldn't always be sexual in nature. Grabbing a breast or spanking an ass on your way out the kitchen doesn't usually say, "I love you and I look forward to amazing sex that blows both our minds."

- Touch should be light and sweet with the intention of enticing rather than being aggressive or obvious.

Don't stop there though. Too often a couple rushes into the bedroom, strips off their clothes and goes for the quickie. While quickies can be a fun and exciting part of a healthy sexual relationship, they shouldn't be the standard.

Both women and men as they age, need more enticement in the bedroom to have a great sexual experience. Plan for plenty of foreplay before you even begin to think about which position you'll be able to orgasm the best.

Later in this guide, you will learn several tips to improve and enhance your foreplay. Be sure to experiment with as many as possible to learn what works best for you and your partner.

# Understand Your Partner's Love Language

Everyone speaks a language all their own. The better able you are to learn the language of your partner, the better you will be able to help your partner have the best possible sexual experience. And the better your partner's experience, the better your own.

While everyone has their own unique love language, it is possible to narrow down what that language is in order to have a better head start on understanding your partner. Gary Chapman wrote a book call "The Five Love Languages: How to Express Heartfelt Commitment to Your Mate." In his book, Chapman talks about the 5 standard languages of love. Every person falls within these five languages with some slight variation but it at least gives a place to get you started.

The 5 love languages consist of:

**Acts of Service** - Individuals strong in this language feel most loved when their partner does something nice for them. This could be taking out the trash without being asked or getting their car washed.

In the bedroom, someone who is strong in this language will find the experience most pleasurable by receiving more than giving. This person is most turned on by how the actual act is performed. Pay special attention to what is being done with this partner.

**Words of Affection** - Individuals who are strong in this language feel most encouraged and loved with words. Statements of how special this person is go a long way.

In the bedroom, be sure to tell a partner that is strong in this language how attractive you find them and when and how they are doing something that makes you feel amazing. The more you can share what they are doing right, the more they'll continue to do that.

**Receiving Gifts** - This love language is all about showing someone you love them through a gift. Remembering this person's special days and bringing them something special is the best way to show this person you care.

In the bedroom, you will find that this partner is most turned on by being remembered at other times of the day. Bring them flowers or a special gift to get their Foreplay All Day juices flowing and a little gift of something sexy and edible or a fun new toy to try out also make a big impression.

**Quality Time** - For this individual, they thrive on how much time you give them. Just being present with the other person is often enough to show them just how much you care.

In the bedroom, you may find that your partner desires more foreplay. Give them the time they are seeking and be extra generous before starting the actual act.

You also will find that Foreplay All Day is crucial for this language. Stop watching TV while your partner is cleaning up. Spend time with your partner without distraction rather than rushing off to get your own stuff done. When you are able to give them more time, they hear that as a true expression of love.

**Physical Touch** - This language is about much more than the act of sex with a partner. Physical touch encompasses holding hands, kissing, massages and much more. While some partners may misconstrue physical touch as just an act leading to sex, others find that this is how they truly feel loved.

In the bedroom, be sure to engage fully with your partner on many different levels of touch. Explore sensual massage, kissing various body parts or even testing out different forms of touch. Try out ice cubes or hot wax (but be careful). Explore different textures and pressures.

This language can often be the most fun to explore in the bedroom. Don't limit your imagination to what you can do.

Truly understanding the language of your partner and making an effort to speak their language is a great way to impress them in the bedroom and keep a great sex life going for years to come.

# Let's Talk

Beyond a few moans and a couple of "oh, baby" shouts, most couples don't talk about sex. This lack of communication leads to boring sex that leaves a lot to be desired. Sex talks should be a part of your regular routine, both in and out of the bedroom. The more you share, the more you can really impress one another.

## The Dinner Conversation

We aren't raised to talk about sex, especially outside the bedroom. However, the value of keeping the sex talk on neutral ground and out of the bedroom allows for an open exchange free of pressure that one partner has specific expectations and immediate needs to be satisfied. It opens both partners up to be more comfortable to discuss options that may or may not be used at a later time.

Having sex talks may be uncomfortable at first. Thankfully, it is probably a bit uncomfortable for both of you so you can help one another through together. You can start out simply by stating that you want to have an open discussion about sex. Start slow and work your way up to the bigger details.

Alternatively, use movies or shows you are watching as talking points. If you see something happening on a show, pause the video and talk to your partner about it. This allows the topic to be more organic and less forced or scripted.

There's no limit to what may be discussed. However, here are a few good questions that may help you get started:

- What is your favorite position?
- What is your least favorite position?

- Are you open to playing with some toys?
- What is something you've always fantasized about but been afraid to mention?
- Is there anything that I do that you would really love me to do more of?
- Is there anything that I do that you are not that wild about?

Feel free to expand from there. This just gives you a few ice breakers.

## The Pillow Talk

One of the best ways to let your partner know what you like is to give them verbal queues. While a subtle moan is a good start, get even more clear by using your words. Don't be shy about telling your partner what you really like or what doesn't feel good. Most humans can't claim to be psychic so the only way they can know is if you tell them.

Every person is built a little different. That means that some positions will feel better to some than to others. Some people are more verbal and like to hear "sweet nothings" while engaging in sex. Others are all about the sensual touch. And to add an extra layer, this can all change as we get older or just explore new things. Being able to communicate these preferences ongoing is what creates an amazing lifelong sexual connection.

Is your partner shy when it comes to letting you know? Don't be afraid to ask. When you show them how important their needs are, you can't help but impress.

# Part 2
# Exploring New Things

# Taking the Wheel:
## Masturbation doesn't have to be a solo act.

From our earliest beginnings, most individuals learned how to self stimulate through masturbation. Perhaps because of this beginning, it has always felt like something that was only supposed to happen when no one else was around.

It isn't uncommon for a man to ask his partner to masturbate while he watches. But why is this such a turn on for men?

First of all, it isn't limited to men. Many women also enjoy watching their men masturbate. Part of the appeal is that those individuals tend to be very visual. They enjoy seeing what their partner does to make themselves feel great in order to learn how to duplicate those moves. This is a great way to learn what it is that your partner really enjoys most when it comes to touch.

In addition, some individuals are highly turned on by seeing their partners in pleasure. Being able to simply sit back and watch allows the individual to focus just on this sight rather than being distracted by what they, themselves are having to do.

Don't be afraid to self stimulate in front of your partner if that is what they are asking from you. You can learn a lot about your own body while also creating an amazing experience for your partner, all while impressing them with your own confidence.

If it feels uncomfortable to do this while your partner watches, ask him or her to join in and masturbate simultaneously. This might help take some of the pressure off both of you. You can each watch while being somewhat occupied at the same time.

You might also experiment with using toys to masturbate in front of one another. There are definitely a wide selection of toys for both men and women. Find one you like and you'll soon forget all about who's watching.

For an extra treat, plan to surprise your partner by letting them "catch" you in the act. Determine when they are likely to arrive home and be fully engaged in your thing when they walk in. Whatever time of day it might be, it is sure to heat things up for the next few hours.

And, as a final thought, mutual masturbation can be a great way to take some of the pressure off when all things aren't feeling just right down there but you still want to have some fun. Don't be afraid to take the wheel and do the driving yourself. You are sure to impress your visual partner by doing so.

# Teasing and Denial

If you haven't been living under a rock for the last five or ten years, you've heard of sexual bondage and BDSM from books and movies like "50 Shades of Grey". While you might not be ready to go all in with a dominate/submissive relationship, there are some great practices from this industry that can truly impress your partner and spice up your sex life.

Teasing and denial is the act of bringing your partner to a heightened sexual state without allowing him or her to reach full orgasm. The human instinct is to orgasm as quickly as possible because of the pleasurable feelings associated with it. Waiting as long as possible to complete this act increases the feelings of pleasure both physically and psychologically.

## True Denial

For most individuals familiar with teasing and denial, it is about the lack of control the partner feels. While this may not sound exciting to everyone, there is a large population of individuals that are highly turned on by not having this kind of control. In this category, denial may mean that the partner is left without a satisfying release for a day or even longer.

This game often works well on dominate types who are seeking to give up some control in their lives. Repeatedly teasing them to the point of orgasm and then denying a satisfying full release time and again will have them eating out of your hands (and anything else you might want them to eat out of).

Just remember, while you can take advantage of this scenario and have a lot of extra focus and attention on your needs, the partner who is turned on by this practice of being denied is also getting a significant benefit. Your ability to take control of the situation is quite impressive to them.

## Just the Tease

The alternative way to play this game and possibly one more pleasing to someone less committed to the control aspect, is that the tease is about a build up to an orgasm that is far more intense than an average orgasm. This usually occurs over one session as opposed to multiple possible sessions for denial.

For this technique, you can use toys or any form of manual stimulation. It is much easier to control the outcome this way than it is through full intercourse. With your method of choice, bring your partner close to orgasm.

Have your partner tell you when he or she gets close to orgasm as they are much better at knowing this than you are at reading their body language. Once you've performed this treat on them a few times, they will definitely be willing to wait and happy to let you know to back off a little. Encourage your partner to try NOT to orgasm to heighten the tension and increase the intensity.

Once your partner can't hold out any longer, allow them to have a full and complete orgasm. The feelings will be much more intense and satisfying after having had to wait and delay.

Whether you want to explore simply teasing your partner into a more rich and satisfying orgasm or they are asking you to take a more controlling role, teasing and denial can bring an interesting and fun twist to your sex life.

# Silly Rabbit, Toys Are For Sharing

Nearly 50% of women own a sex toy and yet, only around 20% of couples use toys during sex. Part of the reason for this discrepancy is due to the myths surrounding sex toys and part of this is simply not knowing how to bring it up in conversation.

Let's first talk about a couple of dominate myths couples believe about why toys aren't for sharing.

**Decreased Sensitivity** - Some people believe that vibrators will decrease a woman's sensitivity to regular stimulation making it harder for her to orgasm without the aid of a vibrator. This has been proven false and women can easily go back and forth between the two forms of stimulation without any decrease in sensitivity. In fact, women are much more likely to experience orgasm with clitoral stimulation than with strictly vaginal stimulation. A vibrator or other sex toy can help facilitate this process.

**Men are Too Sensitive** - There are also some individuals who believe men are too sensitive to have vibrators used on them. While this can be true, it only means proceed with caution to see what the limits are. Most men are just fine having a vibrator stimulate any or all parts of their sexual anatomy.

Now that you've decided you want to move forward with introducing toys into your sexual sessions, let's talk about a few ways you can do this.

**Toy Selection**

First, select the right toys. Not all toys are well suited for couples play while others are designed just for that. Your choices will be somewhat determined by your comfort level as well. If you are interested in exploring anal sex but not ready for the full thing, then a small dildo may be just what you need to get you started. If you enjoy mutual masturbation, vibrators for the women and sleeves for the men might be just the way to go.

For the best possible experience, consider going shopping together (even online in the privacy of your own home) to select something that would be fun and exciting to both of you. Doing the research together can help make the transition to using the toys together that much easier.

**Using Toys**

Now that you have the toys in the bedroom with you, don't feel pressured to be perfect the first time around. Most toys require a little getting used to and that can be part of the fun. Experiment together to see what works best. You may just find multiple ways you can have fun with the same toy!

Now go have fun and play with some toys.

# Change of Scenery

If you really want to spice things up and impress your partner, ditch the bedroom scene. It is far too easy to fall into a rut of sex being that thing you do before rolling over and going to sleep at night. Mixing it up and making sex about, well sex, instead of about an act that you are supposed to do can start with a quick change of scenery.

## Throughout the House

Every room of the house is open to some sexual adventure.

The kitchen can be a great place to explore with food items and turn cooking into a whole new experience.

The living room may provide for some different positions that will truly drive your partner wild.

Go for the stairs if you want to get in some fun with soft ropes and ties or even just a new perspective.

Sex in the shower can bring on the steam in more ways than one. For an added bonus, get a handheld massaging shower head. The massaging jets can be incredibly stimulating.

## Take it Outside

However, don't be limited to what is within the confines of your home. Get really adventurous and take a turn in some of these different locations.

When was the last time you went to "look out point"? Find a nice quiet spot and see just how steamy you can make your car windows. Just watch out for the gear shift and make sure you have the emergency brake on!

What about skinny dipping? While it seems like something that just the kids do, bringing out your watery side can really ignite your passion and fuel an amazing sex life.

Camping out in nature might bring up thoughts of ants and bugs but when you look past that, the experience can be fun and different.

And don't forget the romp in the hay if you happen to be near a barn for this memorable experience.

A change of scenery isn't about what you do all the time. Instead it is about introducing something new and different on occasion. You can't impress your partner if you are stuck in the same old rut.

# The Other "Naughty" Places

When most people think of sexual body parts, they naturally think of the breasts, the vagina, the penis and sometimes the anus. With this mindset, it's natural to focus only on those parts of the body to stimulate a sexual response.

Fortunately, though, there are many other "naughty" places that can be very sensual and often lead to significant arousal. By focusing on these other places, you will show your partner that you are multifaceted and know your way around their anatomy.

Let's talk about some of these and how you can make the most out of each area.

## The Face

Whether it is the lips, eyebrows or the ears, many people are highly aroused by a simple touch or a light massage in these areas. Maximize these locations by beginning foreplay while quietly cuddling on the couch in front of a movie. You can stroke or massage these areas without any indication of what might come next.

## The Feet

While most women are not specifically turned on by having their men suck their toes, they certainly do give brownie points for a great foot massage. Taking the time to rub your partner's feet can help them to reduce their overall stress level and open them up to being ready for what might come next. This is part of what we talked about earlier in making sure that foreplay is all day.

## The Legs

There are two places on both men and women that can be highly arousing.

First is behind the knees. The soft spot in the bend of a leg can often be very ticklish but it can also create a strong sensation that heightens the feelings in the groin region. Be sure not to take this too far as tickling can often be a turn off if taken too far.

In addition to the knees, the thigh area can be highly erotic. Massage the muscles right up to where the legs meet the groin without actually touching the groin area. The closer you get, the more enticing this can be.

Men often think about going straight for the breasts and the vagina. To really impress your partner, avoid these areas until she is begging you to touch her there. Focus on the other naughty places first.

## The Testicles

Women are often afraid to address a man's testicles for fear that they may end up hurting their partner. Don't be afraid to kiss, caress or even lightly squeeze the testicles. Your partner will let you know if it is too much or just enough.

## The Perineum

The perineum is the soft stretch of skin on a man between his testicles and his anus. This location is highly sensitive and can provide for heightened sexual intercourse. Stimulation can be a caress or light pressure.

## The Anus

While you might not be ready for anal intercourse, the anus is full of nerve endings and playing gently with this area is just one more way to explore your partner's sexuality. Even without penetration, using a finger or a vibrator to lightly rub or caress the anal opening can lead to intense sexual feelings. If you are feeling adventurous, consider using your tongue for this purpose.

There are many areas on the human body that are ripe for sensual stimulation. Explore all of them to determine how to best impress your partner.

# Sensual Massage

The sensual massage is about being fully present for your partner. The result does not, in fact, have to lead to sexual intercourse but simply in providing your partner with a truly amazing experience that will entice them to feel better about their own body.

## Preparation

To truly impress your partner when giving him or her a sensual massage, be sure to prepare the room. While it seems cliché; candles, soft music and soft lighting can significantly improve the atmosphere and results. Multitasking and providing a massage while catching up on a tv show is not going to provide for a memorable experience.

## The Basic Sensual Massage

A typical sensual massage involves light touch all over the body focusing on points that will increase sexual energy such as the breasts, vagina and penis. However, the focus of touching these areas during a sensual massage is less about stimulating to complete arousal and more about increasing your partner's awareness of these areas. The touch should almost be more of a tease and a bit of enticement.

## The Energy Massage

Another type of sensual massage is an Energy Massage. In this form of massage, your partner is blindfolded and has on headphones with some relaxing music so there is some form of sensory deprivation in addition to the massage.

Once your partner is ready, the massage begins. However, unlike traditional massage that involves either light or heavy rubbing, a sensual energy massage consists of passing your hands over the various parts of the body without actually making a physical connection.

As you pass over each part of the body, stop and focus on sharing your energy with your partner. Feel the energy pass from your fingertips into their body at each point. You may choose to spend extra time focusing, but not touching, the specific areas of the body where energy is felt the strongest. These areas include the penis and vagina.

It is important to remember that the point of this massage is not to have sex. It is to have an experience with your partner that will allow you both to become more deeply connected to one another.

It is best to perform each session independently rather than back to back. This isn't about taking turns but rather about being fully present for your partner's experience.

It may take a few times to master the art of the sensual energy massage but it can be a freeing and highly enjoyable activity while you are learning.

# Fantasy

Fantasy has a long and rich background in sexual history. The human mind is designed to be creative and part of that creativity is dreaming up new ideas about what sexual experiences may be fun and exciting. Individuals are often afraid to share their sexual fantasies with their partners out of fear or shame. Creating an environment where your partner knows that they come first and are what you care about most will help them to open up to your fantasies as well as to be more willing to share their own.

Not all fantasies are meant to be fulfilled and dreams of a threesome with the model on a favorite magazine are usually not possible. However, there are a great many smaller fantasies that are very possible when openly shared and discussed with your partner.

## How To Bring It Up

The hardest part about fantasy fulfillment may be just bringing it up with your partner. It is usually not best to bring up a fantasy in the heat of the moment. Individuals often feel vulnerable and easily manipulated at these times. Have conversations around fantasies when you are both relaxed but not preparing to jump right into business. Start out with simple fantasies rather than jumping in with your deepest, darkest desires. This allows your partner to get used to the idea of something new and different and they may be much more open to using toys during sex than to a threesome with his or her best friend.

Remember that the best fantasies happen when both partners are willing participants. Not everyone is into the same stuff and some ideas may be a big turn off for others. Listen to one another and have an open discussion. If it doesn't fit for both, there should be no pressure to perform.

Your fantasies might involve role playing or use of unusual toys. You might be thinking about an exciting place or even a threesome. Be open to talking about what ideas you have and see where it may lead.

# Making a Plan

Another common mistake couples make is to fall into the trap of believing that sex has to be spontaneous to really be amazing. A solid plan can actually create a better, more impressive overall experience that comes from a place of thought rather than purely need and sexual desire.

Busy couples may find that "spontaneous" sex becomes quick and forced, almost like you forgot to do something and you need to take care of it quickly before falling to sleep. However, the best sex lives come with the idea that sex is a healthy part of an ideal lifestyle and that lifestyle comes with planning.

Your sex plan might include thinking up where and when you will get together for sex. Deciding in advance can help each person to be mentally prepared rather than exhausted and ready to just get it over with.

You might also consider what toys or games you will play and plant little seeds to create some excitement throughout the day or week building up to the "date". Send your partner little hints about what is coming up. Leave little clues around that makes the plan a bit of an adventure.

Having a "sex date" also helps you to be sure you've taken care of all the necessary grooming and any other distractions (kids, roommates, parents, etc...). This plan removes much of the pressure that causes couples to skip sex altogether.

You aren't likely to go on a vacation without a plan, don't just go through attempting to have a sex life without a plan either. Whether your plan is for an afternoon delight or a long Saturday morning in bed, a great plan can enhance the overall experience and start foreplay once the date has been agreed upon.

# Mission Impossible

Even couples that have an active and healthy sex life often fall into the trap of missionary position on a routine basis. Missionary position is the classic way in which couples have intercourse. Unfortunately, the standard method for missionary position often leaves it impossible for women to have a full and complete orgasm because it is difficult to hit the g-spot region and manual stimulation of the clitoris is often blocked.

## Missionary Possible

Believe it or not, there are actually twists to missionary position that can improve the experience for both individuals. Here are just a few ideas to get you started.

Using a pillow positioned under the female partner's hips can raise the pelvic area to increase sensation to the g-spot.

The male partner can move his legs into a somewhat sitting position to allow for clitoral stimulation.

Both partners can experiment with and alter their movements. Getting into a rhythm together can intensify the overall experience.

## Mixing It Up

Don't limit yourself to missionary position though. Even if you are not the most fit person on the planet, there are many alternatives to try. In fact, this is one area that watching porn videos as a couple can really help you to come up with some new ideas.

You don't need to go all Kama Sutra to explore different positions outside of your traditional tried-and-true fall backs but introducing a few new options every few months can encourage exploration and stimulate new excitement. A few good starter positions might include doggie style, cowgirl or even bent over the bed.

As with many of the other suggestions in this book, don't be discouraged if one or more of the positions doesn't work out for you. The idea is to have fun together and be willing to try new things to keep your sex life thriving.

# The Myth of Mutual Orgasm

Mutual orgasm isn't really a myth. It DOES happen from time to time. What is a myth, though, is that great sex can only occur in the presence of the elusive mutual O.

Pop culture is big on promoting the idea that the ultimate sexual experience always results in a mutual and simultaneous orgasm. Without this, it is just a failed attempt. This myth often leads to misconceptions about what is possible in the bedroom. In addition, feelings of inadequacy result when the simultaneous orgasm isn't reached.

It is possible to increase the chances of mutual orgasm. Men tend to be more able to control when an orgasm is going to happen, therefore, they can estimate their timing a little better. If the male partner allows for the female to take the lead, then mutual orgasm is much more likely to happen.

You will find that many of the tips and techniques we have already discussed will actually improve your results but here are a few more tips to increasing your chances of a simultaneous orgasm.

- Know your partner - When you know what your partner truly enjoys, you can enhance the experience and be more effective with the timing.

- Estimate the timing - Some couples can have sex for an hour or more while others tend to keep it to less than 30 minutes. When you know the typical amount of time your experience takes, you can time things more accordingly.

- Don't be afraid to slow down - Telling your partner you are getting to close to an orgasm and encouraging them to do the same can help slow things down until you both get closer to the actual moment together.

Ultimately, though, simultaneous orgasm isn't always possible. Don't pressure yourselves to feel like sex is only amazing when it does occur. Healthy couples with amazing sex lives often have nights when only one partner will orgasm and other nights when one will orgasm multiple times while the other only has one orgasm. This variety and willingness to allow any of the these scenarios to define an amazing sexual experience is what keeps the sex life thriving for many years to come.

Allowing yourself not to get caught up in what it is "supposed" to look like is the best opportunity to eliminate disappointment when it doesn't exactly turn out the way you had planned.

# In the End

The best way to impress your partner and have an amazing and fulfilling sex life is to build upon a foundation of good communication. Great relationships, both in and out of the bedroom, are based on great communication. The more you are willing to talk to and explore alternatives with your partner, the more impressed he or she will be.

Whether you start small with simple conversations or dive right in to some of the more adventurous techniques in this book, have fun together and you will never go wrong. You can always come back to this book again and again for new ideas and tips as things begin to fall into a new pattern or routine and you want to introduce some new excitement.

Again, congratulations on your desire to improve your sexual partnership and have a healthy sexual relationship!

Printed in Great Britain
by Amazon